MW01228928

KETO VEGAN COOKBOOK
FOR BEGINNERS

Make your Plant Based Meals Exciting in 44 Different Ways by Introducing a Low-Carb, High Fat Keto Diet Recipes Specifically for Beginners

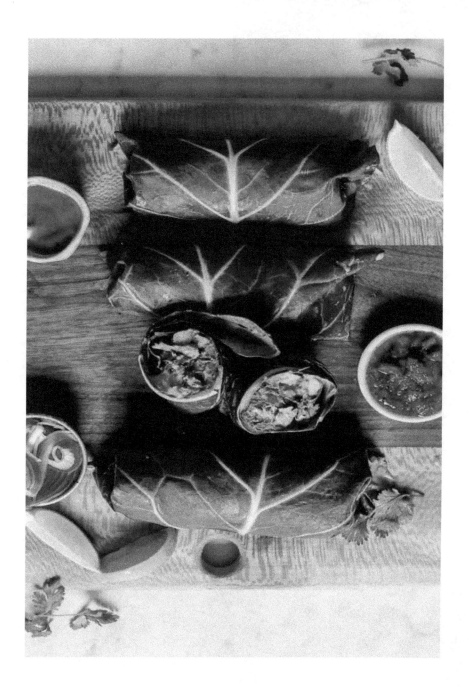

© Copyright 2021 - All rights reserved.
The content contained within this book may not be reproduced, duplicated or transmitted without direct written permission from the author or the publisher. Under no circumstances will any blame or legal responsibility be held against the publisher, or author, for any damages, reparation, or monetary loss due to the information contained within this book. Either directly or indirectly.

Legal Notice:
This book is copyright protected. This book is only for personal use. You cannot amend, distribute, sell, use, quote or paraphrase any part, or the content within this book, without the consent of the author or publisher.

Disclaimer Notice:
Please note the information contained within this document is for educational and entertainment purposes only. All effort has been executed to present accurate, up to date, and reliable, complete information. No warranties of any kind are declared or implied. Readers acknowledge that the author is not engaging in the rendering of legal, financial, medical or professional advice. The content within this book has been derived from various sources. Please consult a licensed professional before attempting any techniques outlined in this book. By reading this document, the reader agrees that under no circumstances is the author responsible for any losses, direct or indirect, which are incurred as a result of the use of information contained within this document, including, but not limited to, errors, omissions, or inaccuracies.

Table of Contents

INTRODUCTION

The vegetarian keto diet is an eating plan that consolidates parts of vegetarianism and keto dieting. Most vegetarians eat creature items like eggs and dairy yet maintain a strategic distance from meat and fish. In the meantime, the ketogenic diet is a high-fat diet that limits carb admission to 20–50 grams each day. This super low-carb admission prompts ketosis, a metabolic state wherein your body begins consuming fat for fuel rather than glucose. On a conventional ketogenic diet, around 70% of your complete every day calories should come from fat, including sources like oils, meat, fish, and full-fat dairy. Be that as it may, the vegetarian keto diet takes out meat and fish, depending rather on other solid fats, for example, coconut oil, eggs, avocados, nuts, and seeds. The vegetarian keto diet is a high-fat, low-carb eating design that takes out meat and fish. Autonomously, vegetarian and keto diets may advance glucose control, weight reduction, and a few different advantages. Both vegetarian and ketogenic diets are related with weight reduction. One enormous audit of 12 examinations showed that those after a vegetarian diet lost a normal of 4.5 pounds (2 kg) more than non-vegetarians more than 18 weeks. Likewise, in a 6-month concentrate in 74 individuals with type II diabetes, vegetarian diets advanced both fat and weight reduction more successfully than customary low-calorie diets. Also, a 6-month concentrate in 83 individuals with heftiness tracked down that a keto diet brought about huge decreases in weight and weight record (BMI), with a normal weight reduction of 31 pounds (14 kg). This current diet's high measure of solid fats may likewise keep you feeling fuller for more to lessen yearning and craving. As a beginner it is not easy to start with keto veg diet but within less time vegetarians may get used to it and enjoy ketogenic veg meals which have low carbs and are beneficial.

Keto vegan recipes for beginners

40+ recipes

1. Instant Pot Vegetable Soup

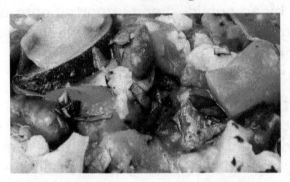

YIELDS: 6 SERVINGS |PREP TIME: 0 HOURS 10 MINS |TOTAL TIME: 0 HOURS 45 MINS

INGREDIENTS

- 1 tbsp. extra-virgin olive oil, in addition to additional for serving
- 1 medium onion, chopped
- 4 garlic cloves, minced
- Fit salt
- Newly ground dark pepper
- 1 tbsp. tomato paste
- 2 c. chopped cabbage
- 2 c. little cauliflower florets
- 2 carrots, stripped and meagerly cut
- 2 celery stems, meagerly cut
- 1 red ringer pepper, chopped
- 1 medium zucchini, chopped

- 1 (15-oz.) can kidney beans, flushed and depleted
- 1 (15-oz.) can diced tomatoes
- 4 c. low-sodium vegetable stock
- 2 tsp. Italian flavoring
- 3/4 tsp. paprika
- Newly chopped parsley, for serving
- This fixing shopping module is made and kept up by an outsider, and imported onto this page. You might have the option to discover more data about this and comparable substance on their site.

DIRECTIONS

1. Set Instant Pot to "Sauté" and add oil, onion, and garlic. Season liberally with salt and pepper. Cook, blending sporadically, until onion mollifies, 5 minutes. Add tomato paste and cook, blending, 1 moment. Add remaining ingredients and mix to join.
2. Lock top and set machine to cook at high pressing factor for 12 minutes. At the point when completed, cautiously turn steam valve to the venting position to deliver the pressing factor.
3. Mix soup and season with salt and pepper.
4. Topping with parsley and a sprinkle of olive oil prior to serving.

2.   Keto Avocado Pops

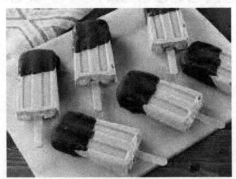

CAL/SERV: 120 |YIELDS: 10 |PREP TIME: 0
HOURS 5 MINS |TOTAL TIME: 6 HOURS 10
MINS

INGREDIENTS
- 3 ready avocados
- Juice of 2 limes (around 1/3 cup)
- 3 tbsp. Turn or other sugar elective
- 3/4 c. coconut milk
- 1 tbsp. coconut oil
- 1 c. keto amicable chocolate (like Lily's)

DIRECTIONS
1. Into a blender or food processor, join avocados with lime juice, Swerve, and coconut milk. Mix until smooth and fill popsicle shape.
2. Freeze until firm, 6 hours up to expedite.
3. In a medium bowl, consolidate chocolate chips and coconut oil. Microwave until softened, at that point let cool to room temperature. Dunk frozen flies in chocolate and serve.

3.   Keto Classic Cheesecake Factory

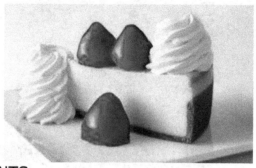

INGREDIENTS
- 1 1/2 cups Graham cracker crumbs
- 1/4 teaspoon ground cinnamon
- 1 1/4 cups of sugar
- 1/2 cup of sour cream
- 2-teaspoons vanilla extract
- 5-large eggs
- 1/2 cup of sour cream
- 2-teaspoons of sugar

DIRECTIONS
1. Preheat the whole thing to 475 ° F. Place a pan crammed with half the water in oven.
2. Made crust: Mix graham cracker crumbs and cinnamon; add butter or margarine. It is placed on the bottom and 2/3 of the man, a 9-piece springform pan chosen with parchment.
3. Make the following: Use an electric mixer to avoid a different, bitter and bitter taste. Blend until smooth and creamy. Scrape off parts of the bottle. View the dishes in a bowl; And get a new dimension. But not until things are known.

Remove something from ourselves and get to work. There is certainly a good choice in a bath. BAK for 12 minutes; turn to 350 ° F once and bake until top of procedure turns golden, 50 to 60 minutes. Remove something to a rack to choose from.

4.   Keto Zucchini Muffins

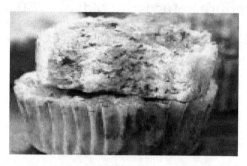

Prep Time: 10 minutes| Cooking Time: 1 hour |
Total Time: 1 hour 10 minutes | Serves: 12
slices | Calories: 166kcal

INGREDIENTS:

- 2 cups of almond flour (click here to see my favorite on Amazon)
- 1/2 teaspoon Kosher salt
- 1/2 teaspoon ground cinnamon
- 1/2 cup granular sweetener (click here to see my favorite on Amazon)
- 1-teaspoon of baking powder
- 2-large eggs, beaten
- 1/4 cup melted butter
- 1 1/2 cups shredded zucchini with skin

DIRECTIONS:

1. Preheat the oven to 350F. Grease a 9x5 loaf pan with butter or cooking spray.

2. In a large bowl, combine the almond flour, salt, cinnamon, swerve, and baking powder.

3. Wrap the grated zucchini in a tea towel and squeeze out as much liquid as possible. Discard any liquid and add zucchini to the dry, followed by the eggs and melted butter. Stir the batter until combined. See notes for adding walnuts, chocolate chips, or blueberries.

4. Pour the batter into a greased loaf pan and bake in the 350F oven for 60 minutes or until a toothpick comes out clean. Let cool before serving. Cut into 12 slices. See notes for freezing, making muffins, and savory bread.

5. Chocolate blueberry clusters

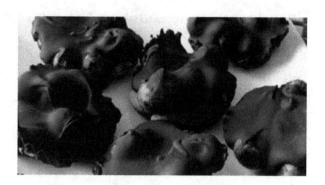

YIELD: 15| PREP TIME: 0 HOURS 15 MIN | TOTAL TIME: 0 HOURS 25 MIN

INGREDIENTS:
- 1 1/2 c. semi-sweet chocolate chips, melted
- 1 tbsp. coconut oil
- 2 c. blueberries
- Flaky sea salt, for garnish

DIRECTIONS
1. Line a small baking tray with parchment paper. In a medium bowl, mix melted chocolate with coconut oil.
2. Spoon a small dollop of chocolate onto the parchment paper and top with 4 to 5 blueberries. Drizzle chocolate over blueberries and sprinkle with sea salt.
3. Freeze until hard, 10 minutes. Serve.

6.   Chocolate Keto Protein Shake

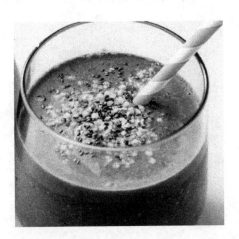

YIELDS: 1 | PREP TIME: 0 HOURS 5 MINS |
TOTAL TIME: 0 HOURS 5 MINS

INGREDIENTS
- 3/4 c. almond milk
- 1/2 c. ice
- 2 tbsp. almond butter
- 2 tbsp. unsweetened cocoa powder
- 2 to 3 tbsp. keto-friendly sugar substitute to taste (such as Swerve)
- 1 tbsp. chia seeds, plus more for serving
- 2 tbsp. hemp seeds, plus more for serving
- 1/2 tbsp. pure vanilla extract
- Pinch kosher salt

DIRECTIONS

1. Combine all ingredients in blender and blend until smooth. Pour into a glass and garnish with more chia and hemp seeds.

7.   Keto fat bombs

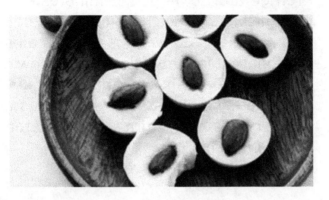

CAL / SERV: 290| YIELD: 16 | PREP TIME: 0 HOURS 5 MIN | TOTAL TIME: 0 HOURS 30 MIN

INGREDIENTS:
- 8 oz. cream cheese, softened to room temperature
- 1/2 c. keto-friendly peanut butter
- 1/4 c. coconut oil, plus 2 tbsp.
- 1/4 tsp. kosher salt
- 1/2 c. keto-friendly dark chocolate chips (like Lily's)

DIRECTIONS
1. Line a small baking tray with parchment paper. In a medium bowl, combine cream cheese, peanut butter, ¼ cup coconut oil, and salt. Use a hand mixer to beat the mixture for about 2 minutes until completely blended. Place the bowl in the freezer to set something, 10 to 15 minutes.
2. When the peanut butter mixture has hardened, use a small cookie scoop or

spoon to make tablespoon balls. Place in the refrigerator to harden, 5 minutes.

3. Meanwhile, make chocolate drizzle: Combine chocolate chips and remaining coconut oil in a microwave safe bowl and microwave at 30 second intervals until completely melted. Drizzle over peanut butter balls and return to refrigerator to harden, 5 minutes.

4. Keep covered in the refrigerator.

8.   Best-Ever Guacamole

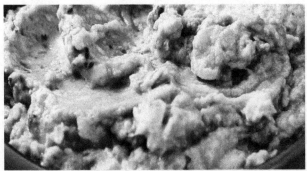

YIELDS: 6 SERVINGS | PREP TIME: 0 HOURS 10 MINS | TOTAL TIME: 0 HOURS 10 MINS

INGREDIENTS
- 3 avocados, pitted
- Juice of 2 limes
- 1/4 c. freshly chopped cilantro, plus more for garnish
- 1/2 small white onion, finely chopped
- 1 small jalapeño (seeded if you prefer less heat), minced
- 1/2 tsp. kosher salt

DIRECTIONS
1.   In a big bowl, mix avocados, lime juice, cilantro, onion, jalapeño and salt.
2.   Stir, then slowly turn the bowl as you run a fork through the avocados (this will ensure the mixture stays chunky). Once it's reached your desired thickness, season with more salt if needed. Garnish with more cilantro before serving.

9. Italian Egg Bake (Low Crab Breakfast)

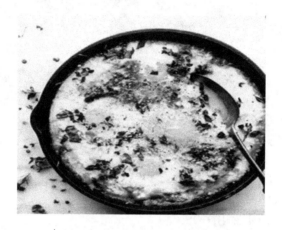

Preparation time 10 minutes | Cooking time 18 minutes | Total time 28 minutes | Yield 4.5 servings

INGREDIENTS:

- 4 ounces of diced pancetta
- 1/2 cup of chopped red onion (about 140 grams)
- 1/2 cup of chopped fresh oregano
- 1/2 cup of chopped fresh basil
- 1/4 cup of unsweetened almond milk
- 2/3 cup grated Parmesan cheese (extra for topping)
- 1/2 teaspoon of chopped garlic
- 1/4 teaspoon sea salt and pepper each (or to taste)
- 1/2 cup chopped fresh tomato

- 1 cup of tomato sauce
- 5 large cage-free eggs
- Red pepper flakes for garnish
- Oregano for garnish

DIRECTIONS:

1. Preheat the oven to 425 degrees F.
2. Fry the pancetta and onion together in an 8 inch cast iron skillet (or oven safe pan) for 2 minutes or until fragrant.
3. Remove from heat.
4. Beat together the almond milk and parmesan cheese. Reserve extra cheese for the topping.
5. Stir in the garlic, tomato, sea salt / pepper, tomato sauce and herbs.
6. Pour the milk tomato mixture over the cast iron skillet (or ovenproof pan) with the onion and pancetta.
7. Using a spatula, make 5 small slits in the pan (evenly spaced) where you can place the eggs so that the yolk doesn't break. Break 5 eggs on top of each crack. If you find you have an egg with a runny yolk, just mix it through the pan, but then add another egg with a solid yolk. Or discard the runny yolk.
8. Add any extra cheese to the eggs and place the skillet in the oven for 15-18 minutes or until the egg whites are set (the yolk softens) and the corners are brown. Baking times vary depending on the oven and the type of skillet being used.

9.   Garnish with Italian parsley and red pepper flakes. To enjoy

10. Keto Breakfast Burritos

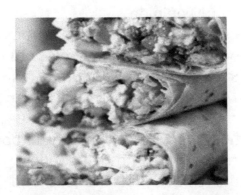

PREPARATION: 20 minutes| COOKING TIME: 10 min | TOTAL TIME: 30 min | YIELD: 6 SERVINGS

INGREDIENTS:

- 6 strips of bacon cut in the middle
- 10 large eggs, beaten
- 4 spring onions, chopped
- 1/2 red bell pepper, diced
- 1/2 teaspoon of salt
- 12 tablespoons of grated cheddar or pepper jack cheese
- 6 8-inch low-carb flour tortillas (I used Ole Xtreme Wellness)
- 6 pieces Reynolds Wrap Heavy-Duty Aluminum Foil , cut 25 x 30 cm each
- hot sauce for serving, optional

DIRECTIONS:

- Cook both sides of the tortillas on a hot baking tray or over an open flame. Keep it warm in the oven if you eat right away. This helps the tortillas get smoother and also improves the flavor in my opinion.
- Heat a large non-stick frying pan over medium heat. Add the bacon and cook until cooked through, about 4 to 5 minutes. Transfer with a slotted spoon to drain onto a paper towel-lined plate.
- Beat the eggs with salt in a large bowl. Stir in the spring onions and bell pepper.
- Discard the bacon fat and let stand 1 teaspoon and add the eggs, let them rest on the bottom and stir several times to cook through, set aside.
- On a clean work surface, spread a generous 1/2 cup of the egg mixture over the bottom third of the tortilla. Top each with a slice of bacon and 2 tablespoons of cheese. Roll from the bottom, fold the left and right corners towards the center and continue to roll into a tight cylinder. Set aside, seam down, and repeat with remaining tortillas and filling.
- If you want to eat right away, heat a skillet over medium heat. While hot, spray the pan with oil and add the burritos seam side down. Cook, covered, until the bottom of the burritos is golden brown, about 2 minutes on each side. Serve with hot sauce or salsa, if desired.

11. Keto chocolate cake

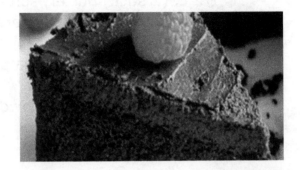

YIELD: 12 SERVES | PREP TIME: 0 HOURS 15 MIN | TOTAL TIME: 1 HOUR 30 MIN

INGREDIENTS:
FOR THE CAKE

- Baking spray
- 1 1/2 c. almond flour
- 2/3 c. unsweetened cocoa powder
- 3/4 c. coconut flour
- 1/4 c. linseed meal
- 2 teaspoons. baking powder
- 2 teaspoons. baking powder
- 1 tsp. kosher salt
- 1/2 c. (1 stick) butter, softened
- 3/4 c. keto-friendly granulated sugar (such as Swerve)
- 4 large eggs
- 1 tsp. pure vanilla extract
- 1 c. almond milk
- 1/3 c. strong brewed coffee

FOR THE BUTTER CREAM

- 2 (8-oz.) Blocks of cream cheese, softened
- 1/2 c. (1 stick) butter, softened
- 3/4 c. keto-friendly powdered sugar (such as Swerve)
- 1/2 c. unsweetened cocoa powder
- 1/4 c. coconut flour
- 1/4 tsp. instant coffee powder
- 3/4 c. heavy cream
- Squeeze kosher salt

DIRECTIONS

1. Preheat the oven to 350 ° and line two 8" pans with parchment paper and grease them with cooking spray. In a large bowl, combine almond flour, cocoa powder, coconut flour, flaxseed flour, baking powder, baking powder, and salt.
2. In another large bowl with a handheld mixer, beat together butter and Swerve until light and fluffy. Add the eggs one at a time and then add vanilla. Add dry and mix until just combined, then stir in milk and coffee.
3. Divide batter among prepared pans and bake until toothpick inserted in center comes out clean, 28 minutes. Let cool completely.
4. To make frosting: In a large bowl, with a hand mixer, beat cream cheese and butter until smooth. Add Swerve, cocoa powder, coconut flour and instant coffee and beat until there are no more lumps. Add cream and a pinch of salt and beat until combined.

5. Place a cake tin on a serving platter or cake stand and spread a thick layer of buttercream on top. Repeat with the remaining layers and then the sides of the cake.

12. Chocolate Covered Strawberry Cubes

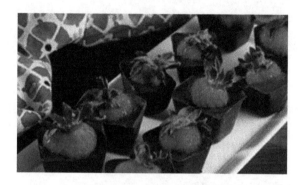

YIELD: 14 – 16 TOTAL TIME: 4 HOURS 10 MIN

INGREDIENTS:

- 2 c. chocolate chips
- 2-tablespoons. coconut oil
- 16 fresh strawberries with stems (depending on your ice cube tray)

DIRECTIONS

1. In a medium bowl, stir together melted chocolate chips and coconut oil.
2. Scoop a layer of chocolate mixture into the bottom of each ice cube tray and cover each with a strawberry, stem side up. Spoon the remaining chocolate mixture over the strawberries.
3. Freeze until the chocolate is firm, 4 to 5 hours.

13. Keto Chocolate Mug Cake

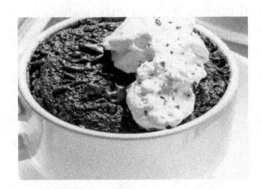

CAL / SERV: 470 YIELD: 1 SERVING PREP TIME: 0 HOURS 5 MIN TOTAL TIME: 0 HOURS 5 MIN

INGREDIENTS:

- 2 tablespoons. butter
- 1/4 c. almond flour
- 2 tablespoons. cocoa powder
- 1 large egg, beaten
- 2 tablespoons. Keto-friendly chocolate chips, such as Lily's
- 2 tablespoons. granulated swerve
- 1/2 tsp. baking powder
- Squeeze kosher salt
- 1/4 c. whipped cream, to serve

DIRECTIONS

1. Place butter in a microwave safe mug and heat until melted, 30 seconds. Add the remaining except whipped cream and stir until completely combined. Cook for 45 seconds to 1 minute, or until cake is set but still fudgy.
2. Top with whipped cream to serve.

14. Baked Keto Bread

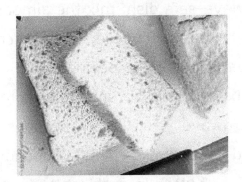

INGREDIENTS:

- 3 tablespoons almond flour
- 1 egg
- 1/2 teaspoon baking powder
- 1/4 teaspoon salt
- 1 tablespoon butter melted
- *optional - 1 tablespoon butter saved for later

DIRECTIONS:

1. In a microwave-safe dish, mix the almond flour with the Parmesan cheese, grated cheddar cheese, sea salt, onion powder, and baking powder. Mix egg and oil until fully combined, then microwave for 90 seconds. It's microwaved and looks like a spongy egg creation! Heat butter in a skillet over medium heat. Let the 'bread' cool for 2 minutes and then cut it in half horizontally into two thinner slices of bread. Fry in a skillet until the bread is nicely toasted on both sides. Let cool for a few minutes before using it for burgers or sandwiches.

15. Keto hot chocolate

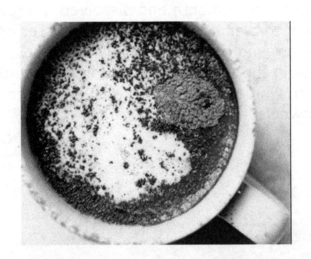

YIELD: 1 CUP PREP TIME: 0 HOURS 5 MIN
TOTAL TIME: 0 HOUR 10 MIN

INGREDIENTS:

- 2 tablespoons. unsweetened cocoa powder, plus more for garnish
- 2 1/2 tsp. keto-friendly sugar, such as Swerve
- 1 1/4 c. water
- 1/4 c. heavy cream
- 1/4 tsp. pure vanilla extract
- Whipped cream, to serve

DIRECTIONS

1. In a small saucepan over medium heat, beat cocoa, Swerve and about 2 tablespoons of water until smooth and dissolved. Increase heat to medium, add remaining water and cream and beat occasionally until hot.
2. Stir in the vanilla and pour into a mug. Serve with whipped cream and a layer of cocoa powder.

16. Keto Pumpkin Cheesecake

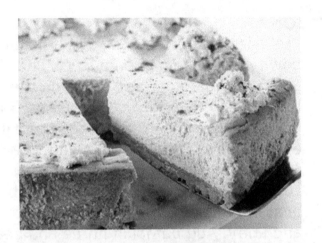

YIELD: 16 SERVINGS PREPARATION TIME: 0 HOURS 10 MIN TOTAL TIME: 7 HOURS 30 MIN

INGREDIENTS:

FOR THE CRUST

- 1 1/2 c. almond flour
- 1/4 c. coconut flour
- 2 tablespoons. granulated swerve
- 1/2 tsp. cinnamon
- 1/4 tsp. kosher salt
- 7 tbsp. melted butter

BEFORE FILLING

- 4 (8-oz.) Block's cream cheese, softens
- 1/2 c. brown sugar Swerve
- 1 c. pumpkin puree
- 3 large eggs
- 1 tsp. pure vanilla extract
- 1 tsp. cinnamon

- 1/2 tsp. ground ginger
- 1/4 tsp. kosher salt
- Whipped cream, for garnish
- Chopped roasted pecans, for garnish

DIRECTIONS

1. Preheat the oven to 350 °. In a medium bowl, combine almond flour, coconut flour, Swerve, cinnamon, and salt. Add the melted butter and mix until well combined. In an 8-inch springform pan, press the crust in an even layer a little down the sides. Bake for 10 to 15 minutes until lightly golden brown.
2. Lower the oven to 325 °. In a large bowl, beat the cream cheese and swirl until light and fluffy. Add pumpkin puree and beat until there are no more lumps. Add the eggs one at a time and beat until well blended. Add vanilla, cinnamon, ginger and salt. Pour the batter onto the crust and smooth the top with a spatula.
3. Wrap the bottom of the pan in aluminum foil and place it in a large roasting pan. Add enough boiling water to halfway the baking pan.
4. Bake until the center of the cheesecake shakes only slightly, about 1 hour. Turn off the heat, open the oven door and let the cheesecake cool in the oven for 1 hour.
5. Remove the foil and refrigerate the cheesecake until it has cooled completely, a minimum of 5 hours and a maximum of overnight.

6.   Serve with a dollop of whipped cream and toasted pecans

17. Keto Gingerbread Cake Recipe

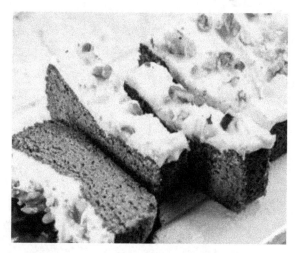

Prep Time: 15 minutes Cooking Time: 50

minutes Total Time: 2 hours 5 minutes

Servings: 10 servings Calories: 275kcal

INGREDIENTS:

- Bread
- 1/2 cup unsalted butter softened
- 1/2 cup natvia
- 1/2 teaspoon vanilla extract
- 4 ounces of cream cheese softened
- 1-large egg
- 1 1/2 cups of almond flour
- 1 1/2 teaspoons baking powder
- 2-teaspoons Ginger ground
- 1-teaspoon ground cinnamon
- 1/2 teaspoon ground cloves
- 1/2 teaspoon ground nutmeg
- 1-pinch of salt

- Frosting
- 4 ounces of cream cheese softened
- 1-teaspoon of vanilla extract
- 1.5 grams of Natvia icing mix

DIRECTIONS:

1. Preheat your oven to 165C / 330F. Add the butter and Natvia to your kitchen mixer and beat on medium speed with the whisk. Add the vanilla, egg, and cream cheese and mix. Add the remaining bread to a mixing bowl and mix. Gently fold the dry into the food processor. Pour the batter into a 9x5in a baking pan lined with parchment paper. Bake in the oven for 50-55 minutes until a skewer comes out clean when you stick it in the center.

2. Let the bread sit in the tin for 15 minutes before placing it on a wire rack to cool completely. Frosting In your kitchen mixer, mix the cream cheese, vanilla, and Natvia Icing Mix. Mix on medium speed until smooth. Divide over the cooled bread and cover with the chopped walnuts. Cut into ten slices and enjoy.

18. Coconut Curry Cauliflower Soup with Toasted Pepitas

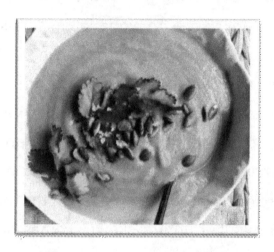

YIELDS: 4 |PREP TIME: 0 HOURS 5 MINS | TOTAL TIME: 0 HOURS 35 MINS

INGREDIENTS

- 1/4 c. pepitas, toasted
- 1 tsp. Additional virgin olive oil
- 2 garlic cloves, chopped
- 1 tsp. new ginger, stripped and chopped
- 1 c. yellow onion, chopped
- 1 c. carrots, chopped
- 1 tsp. legitimate salt
- 1 huge cauliflower head, cut into florets
- 32 oz. low-sodium vegetable stock
- 1 c. full-fat coconut milk (shake well ahead of time)
- 2 tbsp. red curry paste

- 1/4 c. new cilantro, chopped
- Flaky ocean salt
- This fixing shopping module is made and kept up by an outsider, and imported onto this page. You might have the option to discover more data about this and comparative substance on their site.

DIRECTIONS

1. In a little skillet, dry toast pepitas on low heat until brilliant brown, around 2 minutes. Put in a safe spot.
2. In an enormous pot over medium-low heat, heat olive oil. Add garlic, ginger, onion, carrots, and salt. Cook for 5 minutes.
3. Add cauliflower, stock, coconut milk, and curry paste. Mix well, heat to the point of boiling, and afterward stew for 20 minutes. Mix with a drenching blender until smooth.
4. Embellish with toasted pepitas, cilantro, and flaky ocean salt. Serve right away.

19. Keto Long Noodle Soup

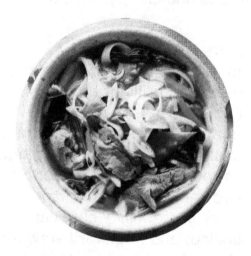

Prep/Total Time: 30 min. |Makes: 6 servings (2 quarts

Ingredients
- 6 ounces uncooked Asian lo mein noodles
- 1 pork tenderloin (3/4 pound), cut into meager strips
- 2 tablespoons soy sauce, isolated
- 1/8 teaspoon pepper
- 2 tablespoons canola oil, isolated
- 1-1/2 teaspoons minced new gingerroot
- 1 garlic clove, minced
- 1 container (32 ounces) chicken stock
- 1 celery rib, meagerly cut
- 1 cup new snow peas, divided corner to corner
- 1 cup coleslaw blend

- 2 green onions, cut askew
- New cilantro leaves, discretionary

Directions

1. Cook noodles as per bundle directions. Channel and flush with cold water; channel well.
2. Then, throw pork with 1 tablespoon soy sauce and pepper. In a 6-qt. stockpot, heat 1 tablespoon oil over medium-high heat; saute pork until delicately browned, 2-3 minutes. Eliminate from pot.
3. In same pot, heat remaining oil over medium-high heat; saute ginger and garlic until fragrant, 20-30 seconds. Mix in stock and remaining soy sauce; heat to the point of boiling. Add celery and snow peas; get back to a bubble. Stew, revealed, until fresh delicate, 2-3 minutes. Mix in pork and coleslaw blend; cook just until cabbage starts to shrink. Add noodles; eliminate from heat. Top with green onions and, whenever wanted, cilantro.

20. Keto Pumpkin Pie

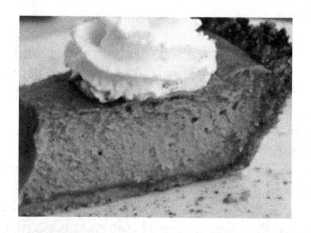

YIELD: 16 SERVINGS PREP TIME: 0 HOURS 15 MIN TOTAL TIME: 3 HOURS 30 MIN

INGREDIENTS:
FOR THE CRUST
- 1 1/2 c. almond flour
- 3 tablespoons. coconut flour
- 1/4 tsp. baking powder
- 1/4 tsp. kosher salt
- 4 tbsp. melted butter
- 1 large egg, beaten

BEFORE FILLING
- 1 (15-oz.) Can pumpkin puree
- 1 c. heavy cream
- 1/2 c. packaged keto-friendly brown sugar, such as Swerve
- 3 large eggs, beaten
- 1 tsp. ground cinnamon
- 1/2 tsp. ground ginger
- 1/4 tsp. ground nutmeg

- 1/4 tsp. ground cloves
- 1/4 tsp. kosher salt
- 1 tsp. pure vanilla extract
- Whipped cream, to serve (optional)

DIRECTIONS

1. Preheat the oven to 350 °. In a large bowl, combine almond flour, coconut flour, baking powder, and salt. Add the melted butter and the egg and stir until a dough form. Press the dough evenly into a 23 cm cake plate and poke holes all over the crust with a fork.
3. Bake lightly golden brown for 10 minutes.
4. In a large bowl, beat pumpkin, cream, brown sugar, eggs, spices, and vanilla until smooth. Pour the pumpkin mixture into pre-baked crust.
5. Bake until the filling wobbles slightly in the center and the crust is golden brown, 45 to 50 minutes.
6. Turn off the oven and open the door. Let the pie cool in the oven for 1 hour, then refrigerate until ready to serve.
7. Serve with whipped cream if desired.

21. Avocado Fudge Cookies

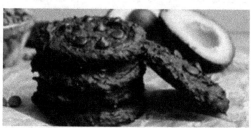

Prep time: 5 minutes | Resting time: 5 minutes | C ALSO time: 12 minutes

INGREDIENTS:

- 100 grams of ripe avocado
- 1 large egg
- 1/2 cup of unsweetened cocoa powder
- 1/4 cup unsweetened shredded coconut
- 1/4 cup of erythritol
- 1/2 teaspoon of baking powder
- 3/8 tsp liquid stevia
- 1/4 teaspoon of pink Himalayan salt

DIRECTIONS:

1. Preheat your oven to 350 degrees F and line a baking sheet with parchment paper.
2. Cut the avocado into the skin and place it in a large mixing bowl. Puree as much as possible with a fork.
3. Add the egg, erythritol, stevia and salt and mix with a hand mixer to a uniform consistency.
4. Add the cocoa, coconut flakes and baking powder and mix again.

5. Scoop 9 cookies onto the baking tray with a cookie scoop. Use a spoon or your finger to spread the cookies out to the desired size.
6. Optionally, cover with lily of chocolate or abraded baker chocolate. Bake for 10-12 minutes, until set.
2. Let cool for five minutes before using.
3. Best store in a zip-lock bag in the refrigerator for up to a week. To enjoy!

22. Greek salad

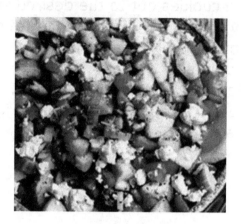

Preparation time 10 minutes | Serve 2

INGREDIENTS:

- 3 (12 oz.) Ripe tomatoes
- ½ (5 1 / 3 oz.) Of Cucumber
- ½ red onion
- ½ green pepper
- 7 oz. feta cheese
- 10 black Greek olives
- ¼ cup of olive oil
- ½ tbsp red wine vinegar
- salt and pepper
- 2 tsp dried oregano

DIRECTIONS:

1. Cut the tomatoes and cucumber into bite-sized pieces. Cut the bell pepper and onion into thin slices. Arrange on a serving platter or, if possible, place the salad on individual salad plates.

2. Add feta cheese and olives and drizzle olive oil and vinegar over the salad.
4. Season with salt and pepper. Sprinkle with crumbled oregano and serve.

23. Keto Zucchini and Walnut Salad

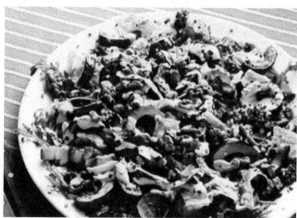

Preparation time 20 + 15 minutes | Servings 4

INGREDIENTS:

- Dressing
- 2 tbsp olive oil
- ¾ cup of mayonnaise or vegan mayonnaise
- 2 tsp lemon juice
- 1 clove of garlic, finely chopped
- ½ teaspoon of salt
- ¼ tsp chili powder
- Salad
- 1 head of romaine lettuce
- 4 oz. (5 2 / 3 cups) arugula lettuce
- ¼ cup of finely chopped fresh chives or spring onions
- 2 (14 oz.) Zucchini
- 1 tbsp olive oil
- salt and pepper
- 1 cup (3½ oz.) Chopped walnuts or pecans

DIRECTIONS:

1. Beat all the for the dressing in a small bowl. Keep the dressing to develop flavor while you make the salad.
2. Trim the salad. Place the Romaine, arugula and chives in a large bowl.
3. Split the zucchini lengthwise and scoop out the seeds. Cut the zucchini halves crosswise into half-inch pieces.
5. Heat olive oil in a skillet over medium heat until it shimmers. Add zucchini to the pan and season with salt and pepper. Sauté until light brown but still firm.
6. Add the cooked zucchini to the salad and mix well.
7. Toast the nuts briefly in the same pan as the zucchini. Season with salt and pepper. Spoon the nuts on the salad and drizzle with salad dressing

24. Keto Peanut Butter Cookies

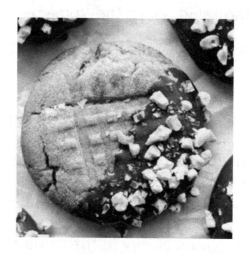

YIELD: 22 PREP TIME: 0 HOURS 5 MIN TOTAL TIME: 1 HOUR 30 MIN

INGREDIENTS:

- 1 1/2 c. smooth unsweetened peanut butter, melted (plus more for drizzle)
- 1 c. coconut flour
- 1/4 c. packaged keto-friendly brown sugar, such as Swerve
- 1 tsp. pure vanilla extract
- Squeeze kosher salt
- 2 c. keto-friendly dark chocolate chips, like Lily's, melted
- 1 tbsp. coconut oil

DIRECTIONS

1. In a medium bowl, combine peanut butter, coconut flour, sugar, vanilla, and salt. Stir until smooth.
2. Cover a baking tray with parchment paper. Use a small cookie scoop to shape the mixture into circles and press down lightly to flatten slightly and place on baking tray. Freeze until firm, about 1 hour.
3. In a medium bowl, whisk together melted chocolate and coconut oil.
4. With a fork, dip peanut butter rounds in chocolate until completely covered and return to the baking sheet. Drizzle with more peanut butter and freeze until the chocolate hardens, about 10 minutes.
5. Serve cold. Store leftovers in the freezer.

25. Magical Keto Cookies

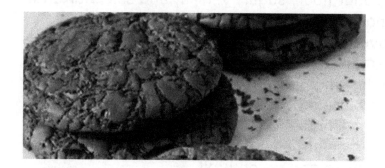

CAL / SERV: 130 YIELD: 15 PREPARATION TIME: 0 HOURS 10 MIN TOTAL TIME: 0 HOURS 35 MIN

INGREDIENTS:
- 1/4 c. coconut oil
- 3 tablespoons. butter softened
- 3 tablespoons. granulated Swerve sweetener
- 1/2 tsp. kosher salt
- 4 large egg yolks
- 1 c. sugar-free dark chocolate chips, like Lily's
- 1 c. coconut flakes
- 3/4 c. roughly chopped walnuts

DIRECTIONS

1. Preheat the oven to 350 ° and line a baking tray with parchment paper. In a large bowl, stir together coconut oil, butter, sweetener, salt, and egg yolks. Mix chocolate chips, coconut and walnuts.
2. Drop the batter onto the prepared baking sheet by the spoon and bake for 15 minutes until golden brown.

26. Chocolate Keto Cookies

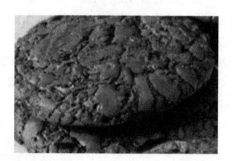

INGREDIENTS:

- 2 1/2 tbsp. butter
- 3 tablespoons. keto chocolate chips, divided
- 1 large egg
- 1 tsp. pure vanilla extract
- 2/3 c. blanched almond flour
- 1/3 c. confectioners Swerve
- 3 1/2 tbsp. dark unsweetened cocoa powder
- 1/2 tsp. baking powder
- Squeeze kosher salt

DIRECTIONS

1. Preheat the oven to 325 °. In a medium bowl, add the butter and half of the chocolate chips. Microwave for 15 to 30 seconds - just enough time for the butter and chocolate to melt slightly. Mix the two until a chocolate sauce forms.
2. In a small bowl, add the egg and beat until the yolk mixes with the white. Once it does, add the egg and vanilla extract to the bowl with the chocolate sauce. Mix again.
3. Add the rest of the dry save some chocolate chips to cover the cookies. Mix until a ball of chocolate chip cookie dough forms.
4. Use a cookie scoop (or a tablespoon) to make 11 even sized cookies. Place the cookies on a baking tray lined with parchment paper and cover each cookie with the remaining chocolate chips. Flatten each biscuit with a spoon or spatula.
5. Bake for 8 to 10 minutes. They should be VERY soft when they come out of the oven, but don't worry, this is normal!
6. Let the cookies cool in the baking tray. When they cool, they will stiffen and become firmer.
2. Once they have cooled, enjoy them and keep the leftovers in an airtight container in the refrigerator.

27. Walnut Snowball Cookies

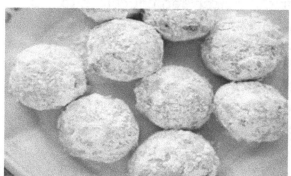

YIELD: 15 PREPARATION TIME: 0 HOURS 10 MIN TOTAL TIME: 1 HOUR 5 MIN

INGREDIENTS:

- 1/2 c. (1 stick) melted butter
- 1 large egg
- 50 drops of liquid stevia (about 1/4 tsp.)
- 1/2 tsp. pure vanilla extract
- 1 c. walnuts
- 1/2 c. coconut flour, plus 1 to 2 tbsp. more for roles
- 1/2 c. confectioners Swerve, divided

DIRECTIONS

1. Preheat your oven to 300 ° and line a baking tray with parchment paper. Combine melted butter, egg, stevia and vanilla extract in a large bowl and set aside.
3. Add walnuts to a food processor and pulse until ground. Pour walnut flour into a medium bowl and add coconut flour and 1/4 cup Swerve and pulse until combined.
4. Add the dry mixture to the wet mixture in two parts and beat to combine. At this point, the dough should be soft but firm enough to make balls by hand without sticking to your palms. If it is not the right consistency, add 1 to 2 tablespoons extra coconut flour and mix.
5. Make 15 equal sized balls and place them on the prepared baking sheet. They do not spread in the oven.
6. Bake for 30 minutes.
7. Let cool for 5 minutes and then roll the (still warm) balls in the remaining 1/4 cup of Swerve.
8. Put them back on the parchment paper and let them cool completely, another 20 to 30 minutes, before you eat them.

28. Keto Pecan Crescent Cookies

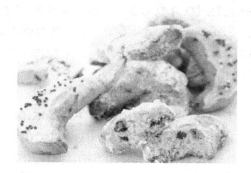

YIELD: 20 PREP TIME: 0 HOURS 20 MIN TOTAL TIME: 1 HOUR 5 MIN

INGREDIENTS:

FOR THE COOKIES

- 2 c. almond flour
- 1 c. finely chopped pecans
- 2 tablespoons. coconut flour
- 1/2 tsp. baking powder
- 1/4 tsp. kosher salt
- 1/2 c. (1 stick) butter, softened
- 2/3 c. Brown sugar swerve (or regular swerve and 2 teaspoons Yacon syrup)
- 1 large egg
- 1/2 tsp. pure vanilla extract

FOR THE VANILLA GLAZE

- 2/3 c. powdered sweetener or erythritol powder
- 6 up to 8 tbsp. heavy cream
- 1/2 tsp. pure vanilla extract

DIRECTIONS
FOR THE COOKIES

1. Preheat the oven to 325 ° and line 2 baking trays with parchment paper. In a medium bowl, combine almond flour, chopped pecans, coconut flour, baking powder, and salt.
2. In a large bowl, beat butter with Swerve for about 2 minutes until light and fluffy. Beat in the egg and vanilla extract. Beat in the almond flour mixture until dough comes together.
3. Shape dough into 3/4 ", then roll between palms and shape into crescents. Place on prepared baking trays.
4. Bake for 15 to 18 minutes, or until just lightly golden brown. They will not feel firm, but will become firmer as they cool. Cool on the sheets.

FOR THE GLAZE

1. Beat powdered Swerve with 1/4 cup cream and vanilla extract until smooth. Add 1 tablespoon more cream at a time until a thin but spreadable consistency is achieved.
2. Spread on cooled cookies and decorate as desired.
3. You can also simply roll cookies in powdered sweetener.

29. Super Food Keto Soup

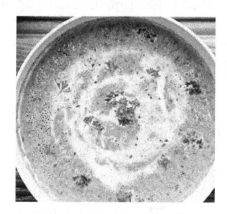

Hands-on 10 minutes Overall 20 minutes
Serving size about 1 1/2 cups/ 360 ml

Ingredients:

- 1 medium head cauliflower (400 g/14.1 oz)
- 1 medium white onion (110 g/3.9 oz)
- 2 cloves garlic
- 1 straight leaf, disintegrated
- 150 g watercress (5.3 oz)
- 200 g new spinach (7.1 oz) or frozen spinach (220 g/7.8 oz)
- 1 liter vegetable stock or bone stock or chicken stock (4 cups/1 quart) - you can make your own
- 1 cup cream or coconut milk (240 ml/8 fl oz) + 6 tbsp for decorate
- 1/4 cup ghee or virgin coconut oil (55 g/1.9 oz)
- ocean salt and ground pepper, to taste

- Discretionary: new spices like parsley or chives for embellish

Directions

1. Strip and finely dice the onion and garlic. Spot in a soup pot or a Dutch oven lubed with ghee and cook over a medium-high heat until somewhat browned. Wash the spinach and watercress and put in a safe spot.

2. Cut the cauliflower into little florets and spot in the pot with browned onion. Add disintegrated straight leaf. Cook for around 5 minutes and blend oftentimes.

3. Add the spinach and watercress and cook until shriveled for pretty much 2-3 minutes.

4. Pour in the vegetable stock and heat to the point of boiling. Cook until the cauliflower is fresh delicate and pour in the cream (or coconut milk).

5. Season with salt and pepper. Remove the heat and using a hand blender, beat until smooth and rich.

6. Serve promptly or chill and keep refrigerated for as long as 5 days. Freeze for longer.Just prior to serving, sprinkle some cream on top. Store in the refrigerator for as long as 5 days or freeze for as long as 3 months.

30. Keto Coleslaw rainbow

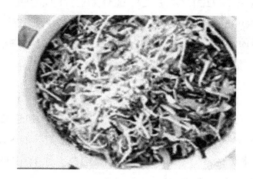

Preparation time 15 + 5 minutes | Servings 6
INGREDIENTS:
- Salad:
- 15 oz. green cabbage
- 15 oz. Red cabbage
- 1 (5 oz.) Yellow Bell Pepper
- 5 oz. Tuscan kale
- 2 ounces. (6 1 / 3 tbsp) Sliced almonds
- Dressing:
- ½ cup of sour cream
- ¼ cup of Greek yogurt
- ¼ cup of mayonnaise
- 1 teaspoon of Dijon mustard
- 1 tbsp lemon juice
- salt and pepper to taste

DIRECTIONS:

1. Using a sharp knife, mandolin or food processor, cut the cabbage, bell pepper and kale as thin as possible. Place them in a large bowl and use your hands to toss them together.
2. Place the almonds in a small skillet over medium heat. Stir frequently until fragrant and light brown in color. Set aside in a small bowl to cool.
3. Place all dressing in the jar of an immersion blender or blender and blitz until creamy and well blended.
4. Pour the dressing over the salad and mix.
5. Garnish with the toasted almonds to serve.

31. Keto Double Chocolate Muffins

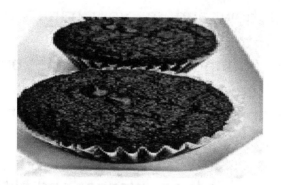

CAL/SERV: 280 | YIELDS: 1 DOZEN | PREP TIME: 0 HOURS 10 MINS | TOTAL TIME: 0 HOURS 25 MINS

INGREDIENTS

- 2 c. almond flour
- 3/4 c. unsweetened cocoa powder
- 1/4 c. turn sugar
- 1/2 tsp. preparing powder
- 1 tsp. legitimate salt
- 1 c. (2 sticks) spread, liquefied
- 3 large eggs
- 1 tsp. unadulterated vanilla concentrate
- 1 c. without sugar dim chocolate chips, like Lily's

DIRECTIONS

1. Preheat oven to 350° and fix a biscuit tin with liners. In a large bowl whisk together almond flour, cocoa powder, Swerve, preparing powder, and salt. Add liquefied spread, eggs, and vanilla and mix until joined.

2. Overlap in chocolate chips.

3. Split player between biscuit liners and prepare until a toothpick embedded into the center tells the truth, 12 minutes.

Nutrition (per serving):

- 280 calories,
- 7 g protein,
- 7 g carbohydrates,
- 4 g fiber,
- 1 g sugar,
- 27 g fat,
- 11 g saturated fat,
- 90 mg sodium.

32. Sugar Free Chocolate Bark with Bacon and Almonds

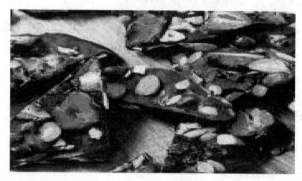

Prep Time: 30 minutes Cook Time: 0 minutes

Total Time: 30 minutes Servings: 8

INGREDIENTS

- 1 9 oz pack Sugar free Chocolate Chips
- 1/2 cup Chopped Almonds
- 2 cuts bacon cooked and disintegrated

Guidelines

1. In a microwave safe bowl, microwave the chocolate chips on high for 30 seconds, mix. Microwave for 30 additional seconds and mix.

2. Microwave for 15 seconds at that point mix one final time. You need to ensure you have a

smidgen of unmelted chocolate chips extra when you haul it out of the microwave.

3. At that point mix one final time and it ought to be totally liquefied.

4. add the chopped almonds to the softened chocolate and mix

5. on a material lined heating sheet, pour the chocolate blend in a meager layer, around 1/2 inch.

6. Sprinkle the disintegrated bacon on top of the chocolate and press in with a spatula.

7. Refrigerate for 20 minutes or until the chocolate has totally solidified. Strip the material from the chocolate and break into 8 pieces. Store in the fridge.

33. Keto Soft Pretzels Recipe - The original low-carb version, delicious!

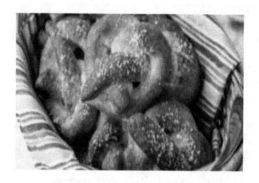

INGREDIENTS:
- 2-teaspoons of dried yeast
- 1-teaspoon of inulin
- 2-tablespoons of warm water
- 5.5 grams of almond flour
- 2-teaspoons of Xanthan gum
- 11 ounces of mozzarella cheese shredded
- 4-tablespoons of cream cheese
- 2-large eggs at room temperature
- 2-tablespoons of salted butter melted
- 1-tablespoon pretzel salt flakes sea salt can be substituted

DIRECTIONS:

1. Preheat the oven to 200C / 390F. Place the yeast, inulin, and warm water in a bowl. Mix well and let rise for 5 minutes. In a large mixing bowl, add the almond flour and xanthan gum.
2. Mix well and set aside. Place a non-stick pan over medium heat and add the mozzarella and cream cheese. Keep a close eye on it as it melts and frequently stirs to avoid browning.
3. Heat until the cheese is thick and pourable. Add the aged yeast and the melted cheese to the almond flour, mix 1 minute before adding the eggs.
4. Mix until a smooth and sticky dough is formed. I recommend putting on food-safe gloves and mixing by hand. Let rest for 5 minutes to rest.
5. Divide the dough into quarters and each quarter into three pieces so that you have 12 balls. The dough is easiest to handle when it is warm and with food-safe gloves.
6. Roll each ball into a long thin block and twist into a pretzel shape. Place them on a parchment-lined baking tray and give a little space with the side as the pretzels will rise.
7. Sprinkle the pretzels with the butter and sprinkle with salt. Bake in the oven for 12-15 minutes. When the pretzels are golden brown, remove them from the oven.
8. Do not burn your fingers if you try to eat them immediately. Let them cool for 5 minutes before enjoying.

34. Low-carb salad of baked kale and broccoli

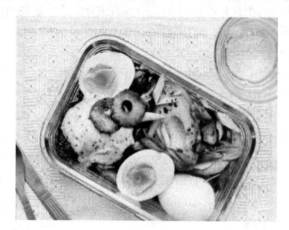

INGREDIENTS:

- ½ cup of mayonnaise
- 1-tablespoon of whole-grain mustard
- 4-eggs
- ½ pound of broccoli
- 4 oz. Kale
- 2-spring onions
- 2 tbsp olive oil
- 2-cloves of garlic
- 2-avocados
- 1-pinch of chili flakes
- Salt or pepper to taste

DIRECTIONS:

1. Combine mayo and mustard in a small bowl and set aside.
2. Cook the eggs however you like: soft, medium, or hard-boiled. Immediately put them in ice-cold water when they are cooked to make them easier to peel. After cooling - divide into halves or quarters. Slice the avocados, remove the stone and slice them.
3. Cut the garlic into thin slices. Heat the oil in a frying pan and fry the slices gently. Remove
4. remove the garlic from the pan and place it on kitchen paper to make it crispy. Keep the oil in the
5. pan. Coarsely chop broccoli and kale. Add a knob of butter to the garlic-infused oil in the
6. pan and fry the vegetables over medium heat for a few minutes until soft.
7. Season with salt and pepper and plate with avocado, eggs, and mustard
8. Mayonnaise. Cover the dish with fried garlic slices for extra flavor and crunch.

35. Salad with keto avocado, bacon, and goat cheese

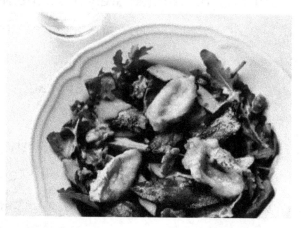

INGREDIENTS:

- 8 oz. goat cheese
- 8 oz. bacon
- Two avocados
- 4 oz. arugula lettuce
- 4 oz. walnuts
- Dressing
- 1 tbsp lemons, the juice
- ½ cup of mayonnaise
- ½ cup of olive oil
- 2 tbsp heavy whipping cream
- Salt and pepper

DIRECTIONS:

1. Preheat the oven to 400 ° F (200 ° C) and place baking paper in a baking dish. Cut the

2. Cut goat cheese into half-inch (~ 1 cm) slices and place in the baking dish. Fry them on the top rack until golden brown. Fry the bacon until crispy in a pan. Cut the avocado into pieces and put them on the arugula. Add the fried bacon and goat cheese. Sprinkle with nuts, use a hand blender to make the dressing with lemon juice, mayonnaise, olive oil, and cream. Season with salt and pepper

36. Broccoli Cheese Soup with Beer Brats (Keto Instant Pot Recipe)

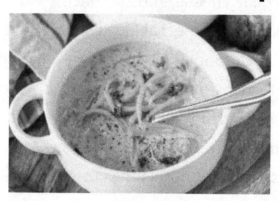

Time: 10 MINUTES COOKING time: 40 MINUTES

Total time: 50 MINUTES

INGREDIENTS:

- 1 lb package of beer bratwurst (regular or cheese is fine too)
- 12 oz low-carb beer (substitute 12 oz chicken stock if desired)
- 4 tbsp butter
- One large onion, diced
- Two cloves of garlic, chopped
- 1 cup fresh broccoli, cut into florets (or 5 cups frozen broccoli)
- / 4 cup (12 oz) chicken stock

- 1/2 teaspoon xantham gum (optional, thickener)
- cup (16 oz) heavy cream or half-and-half
- cups cheddar cheese, grated (medium or sharp)
- 1/4 cup smoked Gouda cheese, grated (any type of smoked cheese will work)
- 1/4 cup parmesan cheese, grated (use only freshly grated)
- 1/2 teaspoon kosher salt
- 1/2 teaspoon of pepper

DIRECTIONS:

1. Select Bake, Medium heat, and preheat your pressure cooker. Melt 2 tablespoons of butter, put the bratwurst in a saucepan, and cook until the roasts are golden brown. Make sure to flip as needed to brown evenly. If the brats don't brown quickly enough, increase the heat to High.

2. Turn off the pressure cooker and pour beer over bratwurst. Secure the lid and select High pressure, 5 minutes cooking time. When cooking is complete, release the pressure naturally for about 7 to 8 minutes, then quickly release. Once the valve drops, carefully

remove the lid. Remove bratwurst and set aside. Keep any remaining liquid in a jar and set it aside in a bowl or other easily pourable container for later.

3. Select Bake, Medium heat, and preheat your pressure cooker. Melt the remaining two tablespoons of butter. Add onions and cook until soft. Add up to 2 tablespoons of olive oil if necessary. If the pan gets too hot, lower the heat. Add garlic and cook for 2 minutes or until fragrant. Switch off the pressure cooker.

4. Add chicken stock, the reserved beer loaf liquid, and broccoli to the pot—safe lid, set on high pressure, and 1 minute cooking time. While waiting, cut the bratwurst into 1/2 "slices. Once the cycle is complete, use a quick pressure relief until the valve sinks. Carefully remove the lid.

5. Remove 3/4 of the broccoli with a slotted spoon and set aside. Using an immersion blender directly in the pan, mix the broccoli remaining in the pan with the stock until there are no more chunks.

37. Turkish fried eggs in spiced yogurt

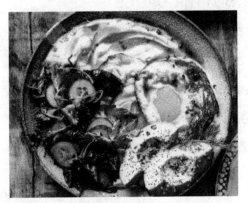

INGREDIENTS:

- 1 cup of plain Greek yogurt
- 1-tablespoon of fresh dill chopped
- 1-tablespoon fresh chopped parsley
- 2-cloves of garlic finely chopped or grated
- salt + pepper to taste
- 4-eggs
- 4-pieces of naan
- zest of 1 lemon
- 1/4 cup sun-dried tomato pesto, homemade or store-bought
- 1-2 cups of fresh baby spinach
- 4 ounces of goat cheese crumbled

- toasted sesame seeds, fresh dill, fresh mint, and salt to serve
- SPICY BUTTER SAUCE
- Two tablespoons of butter
- Two tablespoons of coconut oil
- 1-2 teaspoons ground red pepper flakes
- 1/2 teaspoon sweet paprika

DIRECTIONS:

1. In a bowl, combine the Greek yogurt, dill, parsley, garlic, and a pinch of salt + pepper. Stir until combined. Keep in the refrigerator until use.
2. Heat a frying pan with a little olive oil or butter over medium heat and fry the eggs as desired.
3. Divide the yogurt sauce over a piece of warm / roasted naan. Spoon 1-2 tablespoons of the sun-dried tomato pesto into the yogurt. Then add 1-2 eggs per piece. Sprinkle each piece with lemon zest and fresh spinach. Drizzle the spicy butter sauce (recipe below) over the eggs. Garnish with fresh herbs, sesame seeds, and some crumbled goat cheese. FOOD!
4. SPICY BUTTER SAUCE

5. In a small saucepan, melt with butter, coconut oil, crushed red pepper flakes, and paprika. Drizzle the warm sauce over the fried eggs.

38. Low-carbohydrate slow cooker vegetable soup

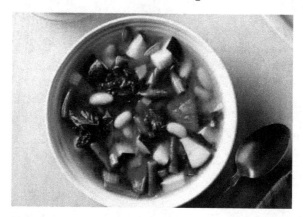

INGREDIENTS:

- Cut four slices of bacon into 1/2 inch pieces
- 2 pounds stew meat cut into 1 "cubes, pat dry
- 2-tablespoons of red wine vinegar
- 32 grams of low-sodium beef stock
- 1-medium yellow onion chopped
- Cut 1/4 cup green beans into 1-inch pieces
- 1-small celeriac (about 6 grams) cut into cubes
- 1/4 cup carrots cut into cubes
- 2-tablespoons of tomato paste
- 1-28-ounce can diced tomatoes
- Crushed 2-cloves of garlic
- 1/2 teaspoon of dried rosemary
- 1/2 teaspoon of dried thyme

- 1/2 teaspoon black pepper, freshly ground
- 1-teaspoon of sea salt

DIRECTIONS:

1. Heat a large skillet over medium heat. Add bacon—Cook the bacon, occasionally stirring, until crispy. Remove the bacon from the pan with a slotted spoon on a paper towel-lined plate. Cover the bacon and put it in the fridge for later.

2. Discard everything except about one tablespoon of bacon fat. Return the pan to the burner over medium heat. Add cubes of beef in batches, making sure they do not touch. Season with salt and pepper. Brown each side of the beef cubes. Do not cook meat. When the outside is brown, transfer the beef to the slow cooker with a slotted spoon. Repeat for the rest of the meat.

3. Once all the meat is browned and in the slow cooker, place the skillet over medium heat. Add vinegar to the pan. Stir and scrape brown pieces until the vinegar has thickened. Pour in about 1/4 cup of the stock and continue to

scrape any browned bits—transfer liquid to the slow cooker.

4. Add the rest of the stock, onion, green beans, celeriac, carrots, tomato paste, diced tomatoes, garlic rosemary, thyme, salt (only when using low-salt stock), and pepper to the slow cooker. Stir gently.

5. Cover the slow cooker and cook on low for 6 to 8 hours. Taste and adjust seasoning before serving. Garnish with reserved bacon cubes before serving.

39. Keto Tapenade Recipe

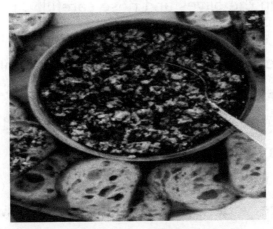

Prep time: 15 minutes |Cooking time: 1-minute
| Cooling: 2 hours |Total time: 15 minutes|
Serves: 28 servings | Calories: 37kcal

INGREDIENTS:

- 11 ounces of pitted kalamata olives
- 2-cloves of garlic
- 1-tablespoon of thyme leaves fresh
- 1 ounce Parmesan cheese
- 1/4 cup of olive oil
- 1-teaspoon of lemon juice
- 1/2 teaspoon erythritol optional
- pepper to taste
- salt to taste

DIRECTIONS:

1. Drain the olives and rinse carefully. Let it dry.
2. Place the olives, garlic, thyme, and parmesan cheese in your food processor and mix at high speed into a thick paste.
3. Add the olive oil and lemon juice and continue to mix for 5 minutes, scraping the side now and then.
4. Taste your tapenade and add the sweetener, salt, and pepper if desired.
5. Mix for two more minutes.
6. Spoon into a container and refrigerate for at least 2 hours or overnight for best results.
7. Serve with a side of toasted Keto Focaccia or Cracked Pepper Crackers.

40. The Best Recipe For Low Carb Keto Yogurt

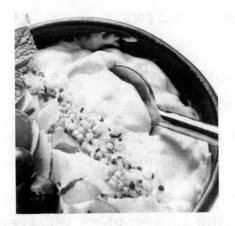

INGREDIENTS:

- Keto Yogurt:
- 1/4 cup of almonds
- 2 cups of water
- 2 cups of heavy cream
- 1/2 tablespoon of gelatin powder
- 1/4 teaspoon liquid sunflower lecithin (optional, for texture and to reduce secretion)
- 2 Probiotic capsules (active cultures)
- Toppings:
- Eaton hemp hearts
- Sliced almonds
- Coconut chips
- Berries (raspberries, blueberries, strawberries)
- Sugar-free jam

DIRECTIONS:

1. Click on the times below to start a kitchen timer while you cook.

2. Sterilize 2 16 oz jars in the dishwasher or with hot soapy water. Dry and set aside.

3. Use the almonds and water to make almond milk according to these (You don't need the vanilla and salt in that recipe unless you want to add them.) Don't use store-bought almond milk - the preservatives will keep your keto yogurt from fermenting properly.

4. Place the homemade almond milk and cream in a medium saucepan over medium heat. Heat gently, occasionally stirring, for 5-7 minutes, until bubbles form around the edges. (Time can vary considerably depending on the material of your pan - mine was a cast iron pan like this one.) Do not simmer or boil.

5. Sprinkle (do not dump) the gelatin over the pan and beat until dissolved.

6. Remove from heat. Sprinkle with the sunflower lecithin and beat until dissolved.

7. Pour the cream mixture into the sterilized jars. Let the jars sit at room temperature for

about 20 minutes until the mixture is below 43 ° C (110 ° F) but still above 100 ° F (37 degrees C). This is critical - a higher temperature will kill the probiotic cultures.

8. Open or cut a probiotic capsule over each jar and stir in the powder. Cover with lids.

41. Fully Loaded Keto Breakfast Parfait

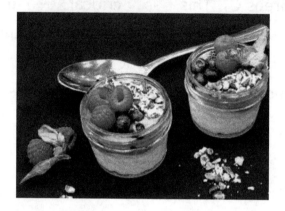

INGREDIENTS:

- cups of Greek yogurt, whole milk
- 0.5 cup of heavy whipping cream
- 6-tablespoons of almond butter
- 2-teaspoons vanilla extract
- 1/2 cup of berries (raspberries and blueberries)
- 4-tablespoons of pecans, sliced
- 2-teaspoons of coconut flakes
- Fresh mint leaves, peeled, for garnish
- Cocoa powder, for garnish

DIRECTIONS:

1. Grab four individual containers of your choice and place them in a prep area. In a bowl, mix the Greek yogurt and whipped cream until fully incorporated. Divide 1/2 cup of Greek yogurt, mix into each container and press down with a spatula to flatten the surface of the yogurt. Then add 1.5 tablespoons of almond butter (or nut butter of your choice), either in the center as a dollop or vertically across the container. You're about to make an Instagram-worthy keto breakfast parfait.

2. Then add 1/2 teaspoon of vanilla extract to each container, 1/8 cup of your desired berry mix (I love raspberries and blueberries) around the container. Top with 1/4 teaspoon of coconut flakes, one tablespoon of sliced pecans, and top with 1/4 teaspoon of coconut flakes. Garnish by gently sprinkling the cocoa powder over the parfait and adding freshly picked mint leaves.

42. Make low-carbohydrate yogurt in the instant pot

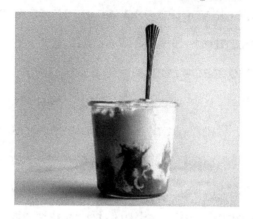

INGREDIENTS:

- ½ gallon whole milk, preferably organic
- Two tablespoons whole milk yogurt with live cultures

DIRECTIONS:

1. Pour milk into the instant pot and close the lid. Press the "Yogurt" button and then the "Adjust" button until "boil" is displayed.
2. You'll want to remove the lid to stir the milk with one hand to heat the milk evenly and speed things up during the cooking cycle.

3. While the milk is heating, fill the sink at least half full with ice water.

4. Once the milk reaches 180 ° F, the Instant Pot will beep to indicate the end of the cooking cycle. Use a thermometer to make sure the milk is indeed at 180 ° F. If the temperature is not up to temperature, restart the cook cycle until the milk is 180 ° F.

5. Place the inner container of the Instant Pot (with the hot milk in it) in the sink with ice water. Keep your thermometer at the temperature of the milking hole until it reaches 110 ° F. Once the temperature has been reached, place the liner back in the Instant Pot.

6. In a small bowl, add the two tablespoons of starter yogurt. Then slowly add 2-4 tablespoons of warm instant pot milk to make the yogurt. Add tempered yogurt to the warm milk in the Instant Pot and stir.

7. Place the lid on the instant pot and press the "Yoghurt" button. Press the "Adjust" button until you are shown a time with the "Normal" light on. Use the "+" and or "-" buttons for your time to set up 10 hours or more. This is

the incubation period for the active cultures to turn the milk into yogurt. A longer time will result in more milk sugar being consumed by the cultures, giving a tarter and low-carb yogurt. NOTE: After you set your time, the display will return to 0:00 and begin counting down until the specified time is reached.

8. When your incubation period is over, you should have a thick yogurt. Place the inner lining in the refrigerator to chill for at least 4 hours.

9. After the yogurt has cooled, place it in a strainer or colander lined with filter paper or cheesecloth over a larger bowl to collect the liquid whey. Squeeze all of the yogurts completely until no more liquid drips. I ended up getting more than three and a half cups of liquid whey.

43. Gluten -free, low-carb biscuit

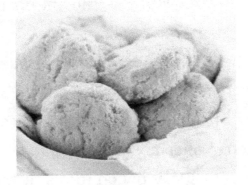

INGREDIENTS:

- 1½ cups of Jennifer's Gluten-Free Bake Mix ™, or another low-carb, gluten-free baking mix (see below for the baking mix recipe), plus a little extra for shaping the biscuits
- 2 tsp baking powder
- Sugar substitute equal to 2 teaspoons of sugar, such as liquid sucralose or stevia
- 1 tsp salt
- 1 cup plus 1 to 2 tablespoons whole milk Greek yogurt (I used traditional Greek gods yogurt.)

DIRECTIONS:

1. Preheat the oven to 425 degrees and line a baking tray with parchment paper. Lightly grease the paper.

2. Beat the baking mix, baking powder, and salt together in a large bowl. Add the yogurt and keep a bit until you see if necessary. Add sweetener and mix with a spatula or wooden spoon until sticky dough forms. If the dough is too dry, add the remaining yogurt.

3. Sprinkle your work surface with some more baking mix. Dip your fingers in the baking mix and divide the dough into 10 to 12 portions. Shape each into a ball and roll to cover lightly with baking mix. Flatten the balls to about an inch thick.

4. Place the cookies close together on the prepared pan. Place on center rack of a preheated oven—Bake for 10 to 14 minutes or until golden brown. Remove from pan. Serve hot with butter or use as a base for chicken-a-la-king, as a topping for pot tarts or cobblers, with fresh strawberries and whipped cream, or to make ham or bacon and cheese

sandwiches. Preheat the grill. Pour the macaroni and cheese into a 20 x 20 cm baking dish (or individual molds). Cover with breadcrumbs and remaining Parmesan cheese and bring to taste with black pepper. Place on the center rack of the oven and grill for 5 to 7 minutes until the breadcrumbs are golden brown.

44. Healthier Mac and Cheese Recipe

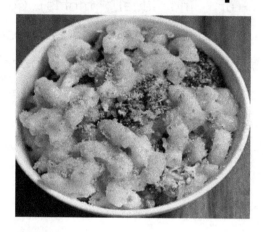

INGREDIENTS:

- 2 cups of elbow macaroni, fusilli, or cavatappi pasta
- 2-tablespoons of butter
- 2-tablespoons of flour
- 2 cups of 2% milk
- 11/2 cups of shredded extra-sharp Cheddar
- 1/2 cup of grated Parmesan cheese (Note: Real Italian Parmesan is called Parmigiano-Reggiano, and its tart, nutty flavor has nothing in common with the stuff you shake out of. A green can. get the authentic version.)
- 1/4 cup of Greek yogurt
- 1/2 cup of panko breadcrumbs

- Black pepper to taste

DIRECTIONS:

1. Cook the pasta just al dente according to the on the package. Drain and reserve.

2. While the pasta is cooking, melt the butter in a medium saucepan over medium heat. Stir in the flour and cook, stirring, for 1 minute. Slowly add the milk while stirring to prevent lumps from forming. Simmer the béchamel for 5 minutes until it starts to thicken to the consistency of heavy cream.

3. Stir in the Cheddar cheese and 1/4 cup of Parmesan cheese and cook until completely melted.

4. Cut off the heat and stir in the yogurt. Add the pasta and stir to coat evenly.

Conclusion

I would like to thank you all for going through this book. All the recipes in this book are for vegetarians who want to have low carb meals and especially for beginners. All recipes are very easy to take a start with Try these dishes at home and appreciate.
Wish you good luck!

CPSIA information can be obtained
at www.ICGtesting.com
Printed in the USA
LVHW011705160521
687588LV00002B/203